THE

DALY DISH

DIARY

GINA DALY AND MR DISH

GILL BOOKS

Gill Books

Hume Avenue

Park West

Dublin 12

www.gillbooks.ie

Gill Books is an imprint of M.H. Gill and Co.

© Gina Daly and Karol Daly 2020

978 07171 9022 5

Designed by www.grahamthew.com

Printed and bound in Spain by GraphyCems

This book is typeset in Sentinel Light.

The paper used in this book comes from the wood pulp of managed forests. For every tree felled, at least one tree is planted, thereby renewing natural resources.

THIS DIARY BELONGS TO:

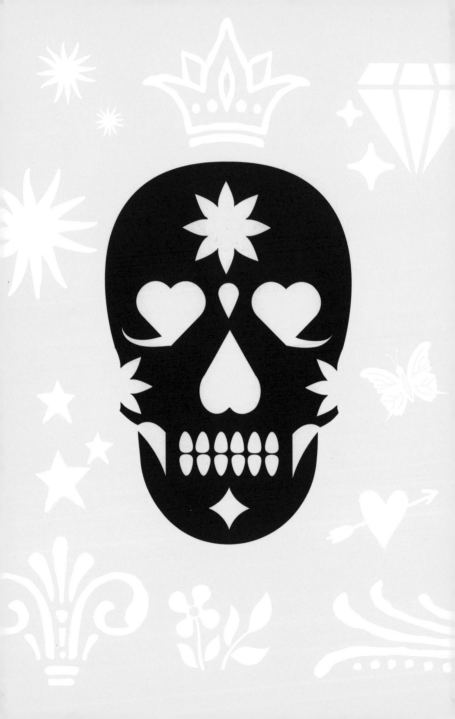

INTRODUCTION

We're back!

Hello, and welcome to this masso diary that's gonna help you keep on top of your daily and weekly food routine and make things a little easier for you. We know you're already bleedin' deadly – this will make you even deadlier!

What worked for us when it came to losing weight and maintaining it ...? Well first off, let's talk about the D-word ... no, not that D-word, the Diet. Some people think: I'll go on a diet and that'll sort me out, and it does and will. But for us, we found that instead of dieting every now and then (which never really worked), we just decided to have a healthy, balanced plan when it came to our eating.

We wanted a lifestyle change and not just a quick fix. We wanted not only to lose weight but to feel healthier in both mind and body. And it's true – when you get into a routine where you're eating better food, you feel so much better in yourself, which will motivate you to stay on track.

Balance being the key here – it's OK to treat yourself now and then. One of the biggest reasons people fall off the wagon when dieting is because they're not eating something they like. Then the cravings get too much and *boom* you're neck-deep in a tub of Ben & Jerry's Choc Brownie ice-cream.

For some people, the thought of making food from scratch can be daunting, but in reality, it's so much easier and it allows you to see and control what exactly goes into what you're eating. It also allows you to tweak recipes as you see fit – you can add a bit more of this, a little less of that, and so on. But it also needs to be exciting and enjoyable and, most important, stuff you actually want to eat. This is where we come in handy!

So, why a food diary? Well, I'm glad ya asked. See, if you use one for your week, it makes it easier for you to keep on top of things and not have to worry about what to be cooking up each day as you've already planned ahead. See? Genius. Obviously, it's a guideline, and if you fancy something different then you can change it up a little.

The great thing about having a planner is that you can sit down at the start of the week and go through exactly what you want to have – basically, building the perfect shopping list. It'll help you stay focused throughout the week and you'll find that once you've a plan in place, you'll be more likely to stick to it. It'll also save you a bleedin' fortune as you'll have less waste and won't be buying the shite you don't need.

WHEN YOU DON'T PLAN YOUR WEEK SCENARIO

There is nothing worse than standing staring into the fridge and not having a notion what to cook. Chances are, if you are tired or not feeling in the best of form because you're jaysus starvin', you will reach for something that needs to be slapped out of your hand. The freezer drawer will be slyly slipped open to see if there're any frozen gems in there that you can just lash on for the kids or the fella, and 'sure I'll just have a little nibble on that and I'll be more organised tomorrow'. Then your tomorrow turns into a 48-hour food bender, and before you know it, you'll be the 'sure I'll get back to it on Monday' person and next thing it's six months later and you are standing in front of the mirror in your granny knickers (nothing wrong with them, I love me aul' granny pants, but I wear them by choice, not necessity, lol!) wondering what the f**k just happened!

Trust me, we've been there (minus the granny knickers for Karol) more than once, and we ain't going back there again!

WHAT WE DO
AND HOW WE PLAN

It's all well and good sitting down with your new shiny planner and your brand-new pen, full of great intentions, until you start asking: How the f**k do I plan a week? What will I actually eat? How do I know what I need or don't need? Relax, don't panic – let us talk you through what *we* do, and it might make things a bit easier to follow.

We sit down on a Sunday (or the night before your shopping day) with a cuppa and pick a full list of what we'd like to cook for the week ahead. We choose breakfasts, lunches and dinners from our book and our Instagram feed, and then add a few new ideas.

Then, we write out all the ingredients, starting with:
1 The meat
2 The veg
3 The spices and herbs
4 The pasta, the rice and the spuds
5 The sauces

We have a nosey through the fridge and presses to see what we already have, then tick the things we need, and off we go to the shop, only buying *what* we need. Trust me, you'll save a fortune, and you'll also be less likely to find a tin of beans from 1965 in the back of your press because the other 25 tins you didn't need were hiding it!

GET INSPIRED

We all want to eat the food we love, but it's hard when they are deep-fried and dripping in grease. We absolutely love watching American food shows and take so much inspiration from some of the dishes we see, but obviously they aren't going to do us any favours. So we work out how we can tweak them, how we can still get the same taste, but without the bang of a deep-fat fryer creeping up the stairs and stinking out the gaff (you know the smell I mean, the one that lingers for days and no amount of Febreze or scented candles is getting rid of it).

You will be so surprised at what you can rustle up when you just have a little inspo. You'll feel like a domestic god/dess and it will become second nature in no time to produce healthier, tastier meals that all the family will love too!

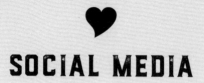

SOCIAL MEDIA

Social media is a deadly place, in both terms of the word! It's wonderful to find accounts that inspire and motivate you, but at the same time, it can have a big effect on you, especially if you are not feeling great in yourself or just having a shitty day.

Make sure you follow accounts that drive you, motivate you and inspire you! Not accounts that drive you to drink, motivate you not to get out of your PJs for the day and inspire you to pull your eyes out because their life is shiny and sparkly and they have no cares or worries and not a chin hair to be seen!

Always remember that the grass isn't always greener on the other side, and what you see on social media isn't always the case in real life. It's very easy to paint a picture for the world to see. Concentrate on you and your happiness, and don't get caught up in other people. You are who you are, and you are feckin' deadly, chin hairs n'all!

MOVING
AND GROOVING

Staying active is a must: you eat, you move, you drink water. Three simple steps to keeping the balance. Not only is it good for the body, but by jaysus it's good for the mind! Now, we are by no means fitness-mad, and I've been to the gym once (that's a story for another day), but we try to inject as much activity into our 'Daly' routine as we can.

WALKING

The cheapest and easiest way to stay active! It costs nothing and you will feel great after a brisk walk! Great for the body, mind and soul. Lash on your headphones, find a banging playlist or podcast and walk the little legs off yourself.

KETTLEBELLS

We inherited a few kettlebells and they sat as little ornaments in the hallway for a while (not gonna lie, like). Then Karol found a chap doing a routine online and knowing what to actually do with them and having a guide made it more appealing to pick them up and give them a bash!

THE LOO RUN

I know, I know, you are going to think I'm mad, but honestly, this is something I always do, especially on days I can't get out for a walk. So, when I need to go to the loo (obviously not when it's a 999 situation), I use the one upstairs, then I run up and down the stairs a few times. You can do this no matter where your loo is in the house. Even if I've to grab something upstairs for the kids, I leg it up and down a few times before I get what I need. Sometimes I end up never getting what I went up for because by the time I've finished, I've forgotten what it was in the first place! If you've been drinking your water, that loo run will quickly accumulate into a rake of steps that you wouldn't have got in otherwise.

SKIPPING

Skipping is an unreal way to get active. I absolutely love it, even if me diddies don't. It gets the heart pumpin' and after 15 minutes I do genuinely feel like Rocky Balboa.

HOOLA-HOOPING

This is a touchy subject for me. If you follow me on Instagram and have seen my attempt at this, you will know why! I really wish I could do it, but I was pure shite ... but that being said, if you have hips that don't let you down, and you can get into the rhythm of it, it really works to tone and shape the body. Alas, for me ... let's just say 'I will in me hoop!'

SNACKS AND TREATS

(AND THINGS WE ARE AFRAID TO USE OUR CALORIES ON)

This is the only part of my day I don't plan, as some days I feel like a snack and some days I just don't! I'm not really a snacker, if I'm honest, as I'm that girl who uses her extra calories in her meals ... Lord forgive me!

Some people say, 'Why would you use that sauce when you could save the calories and make it with a bit of yoghurt and a sprinkle of dust?' (C'mere to me, no one will ever convince me that a homemade garlic sauce made with air and water is better than a shop-bought one.) The little bit we use is really not going to add eight pounds to your arse at the end of the week, c'mon now! I'm not saying to lather every meal in lashings of ketchup, or to spoon-feed yourself straight from the bottle – just use your common sense and don't be afraid to have a little drizzle of sauce!

I do like a sweet hit, which I usually lash into my brekkie – some people see this as a total waste of a good bit of chocolate! If you are inclined to graze, try to buy things like watermelon, strawberries and other fresh fruit. If you like yoghurts, they are handy to have to hand too and you can add in your berries if you need a quick snack.

Now, I'm under no illusion that these are going to give you the satisfaction of a bar of chocolate or a packet of crisps. If you really feel like you want the chocolate or the crisps, just have them. But make sure to keep a few snack-sized packs in the press (I usually pick up the bags that are 99 calories) – just don't eat a share-sized bag all to yourself (which was always my downfall)! Don't buy share-sized bars and say, 'Oh I'll only have three squares on Monday and then I'll have another two squares next Wednesday,' that's just not going to happen! Buy smaller bars, try to keep them under 120 calories, dip them in your tea and enjoy the sweet hit you need.

SHOPPING LIST AND ESSENTIAL BITS

This is a list of some of the most prized possessions in our presses. These are the things we literally cannot live without, and we feel like we could make anything with them when the shelves are fully stocked. Even on the day before we do the shopping, when there's only a scaldy carrot and a packet of ham in the fridge, we'll always find something from these essentials that will make a masso meal.

TINNED BITS
- Tomatoes
- Baked beans
- Spaghetti hoops
- Mushy peas
- Chickpeas
- Kidney beans
- Sweetcorn
- Light coconut milk
- Mustard powder
- Tinned soup (handy to make sauces from or jazz up for a meal)

BOTTLES AND JARS
- Passata
- Soy sauce
- Hot sauce
- Buffalo hot sauce
- Worcestershire sauce
- Black bean concentrate
- Dijon mustard
- Low-fat vinaigrette
- Light Caesar dressing
- Lighter-than-light mayo
- Peanut butter

STOCK CUBES
An everyday essential and the base for most of our sauces and soups. We prefer stock pots, but cubes are just as good.
- Vegetable
- Beef
- Chicken
- Herb

DRIED BITS

- Pasta
- Rice
- Vermicelli noodles
- Egg noodles
- Sesame seeds (deadly for garnishing)
- Instant mashed potato
- Panko breadcrumbs

HERBS AND SPICES

These are the main herbs and spices we use in nearly all of our dishes. We can literally make anything with these bad boys:

- Lemon pepper
- Smoked paprika
- Paprika
- Garlic powder
- Ground ginger
- Chilli powder
- Mixed herbs
- Sage
- Cumin
- Cinnamon
- Curry powder
- Five spice
- Thai 7 spice
- Southern fried chicken seasoning
- Sea salt
- Black pepper

BREAD AND WRAPS

- Wholemeal burger buns
- High-fibre wholemeal bread
- Wholemeal pitta breads
- Wholemeal wraps

OTHER BITS

- Low-calorie spray oil (I use rapeseed two-calorie spray)
- Porridge oats
- Baking powder
- Cornflour
- Cocoa powder
- Vanilla essence
- Vinegar
- Zero-calorie syrups
- Zero-sugar cola
- Zero-sugar orange
- Zero-sugar cordial

YOU'RE
ONLY

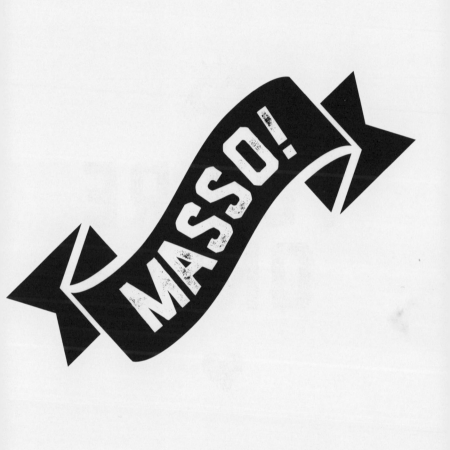

DAILY DIARY

Here's an example of how a typical fortnight looks for us. You will find all these recipes in our book, *The Daly Dish*. We have also included some new deadly dishes in this diary and the rest you will find on our Instagram page in the highlights. No shortage of amazing food to keep you full, satisfied and feeling masso!

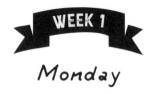

Monday

BREAKFAST

Turkish delight porridge
with fresh berries (page 203)

LUNCH

Tuna sweetcorn & pasta salad
(page 221)

DINNER

Chicken satay
with boiled rice & veggies
(satay sauce on page 129, make extra for tomorrow)

SNACKS

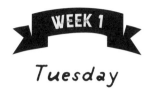

Tuesday

BREAKFAST

Overnight oats

LUNCH

Satay noodle salad

(page 165, use leftover sauce)

DINNER

Veggie / beef lasagne

(page 176, The Daly Dish)

SNACKS

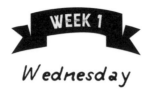

Wednesday

BREAKFAST

Poached egg on toast

LUNCH

Leftover lasagne

DINNER

Me Ma's chicken curry

(page 16, The Daly Dish)

SNACKS

Thursday

BREAKFAST

Weetabix with berries

LUNCH

Caesar salad

DINNER

Beef bulgogi
(page 28, The Daly Dish)

SNACKS

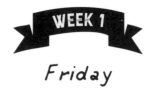

Friday

BREAKFAST

Breakfast pancakes with fresh fruit

(page 196, The Daly Dish)

LUNCH

Rockin' Rueben salad

(page 119, The Daly Dish)

DINNER

Fake-make crispy chicken
burgers, salad and chips

(page 48 (chicken) and page 44 (chips), The Daly Dish)

SNACKS

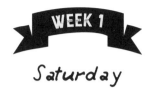

Saturday

BREAKFAST

Sausage and egg muffin
with dishy hash browns

(pages 101 and 102, The Daly Dish)

LUNCH

Light snack, fresh fruit

DINNER

Wild mushroom pasta (page 119)

SNACKS

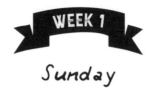

Sunday

BREAKFAST

Bacon, beans and mushrooms

LUNCH

On-the-pan cheese toastie

DINNER

Roast dinner with all the trimmings

SNACKS

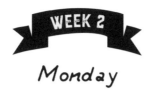

Monday

BREAKFAST

Porridge, jazz it up ta f**k
(page 203)

LUNCH

Buffalo chicken salad

DINNER

Cottage pie (page 33, The Daly Dish)

SNACKS

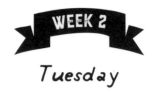

Tuesday

BREAKFAST

Weetabix with fresh fruit

LUNCH

Leftover cottage pie

DINNER

Loaded omelette, fill her up
with veg and a sprinkle of cheese

SNACKS

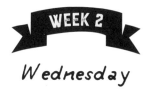

Wednesday

BREAKFAST

Poached egg with asparagus

LUNCH

On-the-pan cheese toastie

DINNER

Chicken and veg stir fry
with noodles

SNACKS

Thursday

BREAKFAST

Beans, mushrooms and toast

LUNCH

Salad bowl

DINNER

Chicken/beef burrito

(page 30, The Daly Dish)

SNACKS

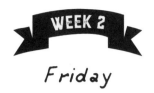

Friday

BREAKFAST

Scrambled egg, bacon, grilled tomatoes

LUNCH

Sambo/toastie

DINNER

Fajita Friday
(page 34, The Daly Dish)

SNACKS

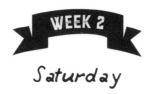

Saturday

BREAKFAST

Waffles with fresh fruit

LUNCH

Spicy tomato soup
(page 127, The Daly Dish)

DINNER

Homemade cheeseburger salad

SNACKS

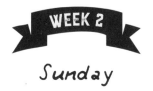

Sunday

BREAKFAST

Dippy egg, mushrooms and soldiers

LUNCH

Leftover spicy tomato soup

DINNER

Chicken, leek and chorizo pie

(page 13, The Daly Dish)

SNACKS

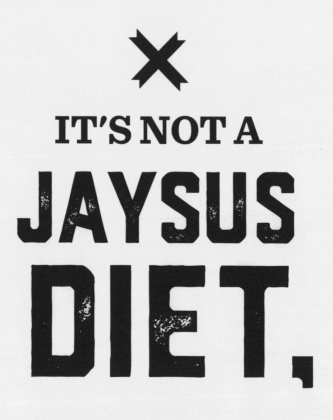

IT'S NOT A

JAYSUS

DIET,

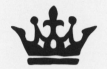

IT'S A

JAYSUS LIFE- STYLE

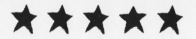

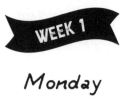

WEEK 1

Monday

BREAKFAST

LUNCH

DINNER

SNACKS

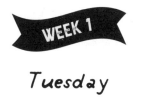

Tuesday

BREAKFAST

LUNCH

DINNER

SNACKS

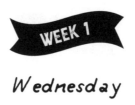

Wednesday

BREAKFAST

LUNCH

DINNER

SNACKS

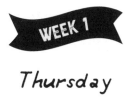

Thursday

BREAKFAST

LUNCH

DINNER

SNACKS

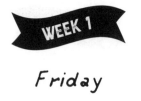

WEEK 1

Friday

BREAKFAST

LUNCH

DINNER

SNACKS

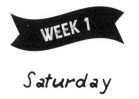

Saturday

BREAKFAST

LUNCH

DINNER

SNACKS

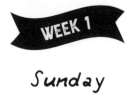

Sunday

BREAKFAST

LUNCH

DINNER

SNACKS

Banana & Blueberry
PANCAKES

My love of banana pancakes comes from when I was backpacking in Thailand in my early 20s. One of their staple breakfast dishes was banana pancakes, and they were epic – I lived off them for months. Here's my healthier take on them with a little added blueberry for an extra flavour hit.

MAKES 2 PANCAKES

1 banana

40g blueberries

2 eggs

40g porridge oats

50ml low-fat milk

1 tsp sweetener

2–3 drops of vanilla essence

low-calorie spray oil

METHOD

Chop your banana into nice chunky slices and set aside with your blueberries. You're gonna make two pancakes, so split your bananas and blueberries into two equal piles.

Pop your eggs, oats, milk, sweetener and vanilla essence into a blender and blast until you have a nice smooth batter.

Spray a little oil into your pan and get it on a medium heat. Pour half the batter mix into the pan, and scatter one pile of banana and blueberries evenly on top.

Cook for a couple of minutes on a medium heat before flipping the pancake over to cook the other side.

Repeat for the second pancake, serve up and enjoy. Drizzle a little maple syrup on top for some extra flavour.

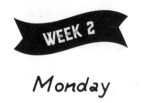

Monday

BREAKFAST

LUNCH

DINNER

SNACKS

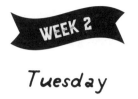

Tuesday

BREAKFAST

LUNCH

DINNER

SNACKS

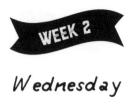

WEEK 2

Wednesday

BREAKFAST

LUNCH

DINNER

SNACKS

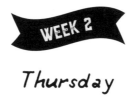

Thursday

BREAKFAST

LUNCH

DINNER

SNACKS

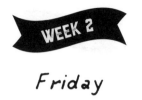

Friday

BREAKFAST

LUNCH

DINNER

SNACKS

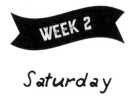

Saturday

BREAKFAST

LUNCH

DINNER

SNACKS

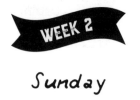

WEEK 2

Sunday

BREAKFAST

LUNCH

DINNER

SNACKS

BBQ Bacon
PIZZA WRAP

You want a quick, easy and tasty lunch? Well, look no further.
You cannot beat a pizza wrap, so yummy, bursting with
flavour and always a favourite with the whole family.

SERVES 1

2 to 3 lean bacon
medallions

1 wholemeal wrap

2 tbsp BBQ sauce
(whichever brand you
prefer)

25g light mozzarella

25g Cheddar cheese

5 mushrooms

½ an onion

METHOD

Get your bacon on the pan and cook it
up to your liking. Once cooked, chop into
small pieces and put to the side. Don't be
sneaking any bites of it – you'll ruin your
appetite.

Get your wrap and dollop that BBQ sauce
on top. Using the curved side of the spoon,
spread the sauce evenly across the base.

Sprinkle the mozzarella and Cheddar
evenly over the base. Finely slice your
mushroom and onion and add them
next, spreading everything evenly. Pop
your bacon on and then place under a
preheated grill for 5 to 6 minutes.

Once cooked, pop onto a serving board
and slice up, or even just roll it up and
munch away.

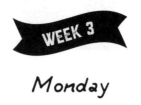

Monday

BREAKFAST

LUNCH

DINNER

SNACKS

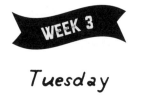

Tuesday

BREAKFAST

LUNCH

DINNER

SNACKS

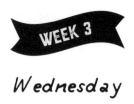

Wednesday

BREAKFAST

LUNCH

DINNER

SNACKS

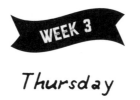

WEEK 3

Thursday

BREAKFAST

LUNCH

DINNER

SNACKS

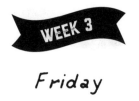

WEEK 3

Friday

BREAKFAST

LUNCH

DINNER

SNACKS

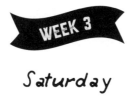

Saturday

BREAKFAST

LUNCH

DINNER

SNACKS

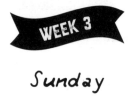

WEEK 3

Sunday

BREAKFAST

LUNCH

DINNER

SNACKS

Alassio Massio
SALAD

What a name for a salad, right? Well, there's a story behind the name. A few years ago, we were on a family holiday in Alassio, Italy. We were staying right on the beach and right beside where were staying there was an awesome café where we ate lunch by the sea most days. One of our favourite dishes was their signature salad, so this is our take on it.

SERVES 2

1 head of iceberg lettuce

handful of rocket leaves

6–8 fresh basil leaves

1 ball of light fresh mozzarella

8–10 small vine tomatoes

1 tin of tuna

150g prawns, cooked and peeled

sprinkle of pine nuts

light vinaigrette

salt and pepper, to taste

METHOD

We're making two salads here (halve the above for one) so get two bowls ready. Start by washing and finely chopping your lettuce and add to the bowls. Follow that with your rocket and basil – no need to chop too much – and then add to the lettuce.

Slice your mozzarella ball into thin pieces and add on top of the salad. Then slice the tomatoes in two and add. Next up, spread the tuna evenly over the top and follow up with the prawns. Sprinkle over a few pine nuts, drizzle some vinaigrette and add a little salt and pepper.

Boom, you have a masso salad, enjoy.

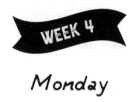

Monday

BREAKFAST

LUNCH

DINNER

SNACKS

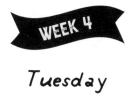

Tuesday

BREAKFAST

LUNCH

DINNER

SNACKS

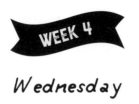

WEEK 4

Wednesday

BREAKFAST

LUNCH

DINNER

SNACKS

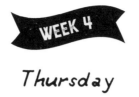

Thursday

BREAKFAST

LUNCH

DINNER

SNACKS

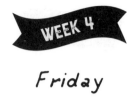

WEEK 4

Friday

BREAKFAST

LUNCH

DINNER

SNACKS

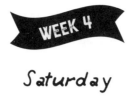

WEEK 4

Saturday

BREAKFAST

LUNCH

DINNER

SNACKS

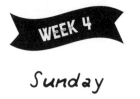

WEEK 4

Sunday

BREAKFAST

LUNCH

DINNER

SNACKS

Winner Winner

CHICKEN...STEW

There's nothing quite as comforting as a warm bowl of stew on a cold winter's night, or any night to be honest. This recipe is guaranteed to fill the hungriest of tummies.

SERVES 2

2 chicken fillets

500g baby potatoes, washed and halved

2–3 carrots, peeled and chopped

1 large onion, peeled and chopped

1–2 tsp olive oil

2 tbsp flour

handful of frozen peas

350ml chicken stock

350ml herb stock

½ tsp turmeric

½ tsp garlic powder

METHOD

Pop your chicken fillets in a pot of boiling water, reduce heat and simmer for 25–30 minutes. Remove from the pot and shred them up.

Get a pot on a medium heat and add your olive oil and onions. Let them sweat off for a couple of minutes. Add your chicken and give it a good stir for a couple of minutes. Then add the flour and mix it all together.

Next up, add your stock, spuds and veg. Stir everything on a medium heat, adding your turmeric and garlic powder.

Leave to simmer for 30 to 40 minutes, and if the stew needs thickening, add a ½ teaspoon of cornflour with a drop of water.

Pop into bowls and serve with some warm crusty bread.

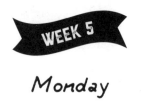

WEEK 5

Monday

BREAKFAST

LUNCH

DINNER

SNACKS

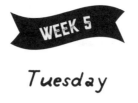

Tuesday

BREAKFAST

LUNCH

DINNER

SNACKS

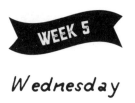

Wednesday

BREAKFAST

LUNCH

DINNER

SNACKS

Thursday

BREAKFAST

LUNCH

DINNER

SNACKS

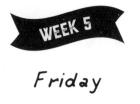

WEEK 5

Friday

BREAKFAST

LUNCH

DINNER

SNACKS

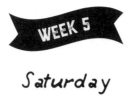

WEEK 5

Saturday

BREAKFAST

LUNCH

DINNER

SNACKS

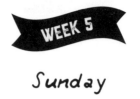

WEEK 5

Sunday

BREAKFAST

LUNCH

DINNER

SNACKS

Curry Cheese
SAUCE

Cheese sauce! Nuff said! This will be my legacy. It will be forever known as Gina's cheese sauce and has adorned thousands of burgers, spicebags, hotdogs and even popcorn (I kid you not) over the years. If you haven't made it yet, here is a little tasty twist on it. And if you haven't tried curry with cheese, you really haven't lived.

SERVES 1-2

3 light cheese singles
50–100ml water
1 tsp curry or curry sauce powder

METHOD

In a little pot, add in the cheese singles and water.

Let the cheese melt over a low heat and blend with the water. Don't worry, it might look a little funny, but stick with it until it becomes blended and smooth. *

Add in the curry powder and that's it. So simple and so tasty! Pour over a masso spice bag (page 70, *The Daly Dish*).

*To note, as this is a slim version, no other oils or fats are added so the sauce will not stay runny as it cools. The trick is to get it into you as fast as you can, but there won't be any problem cause one taste and you'll be hoovering it up!

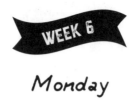

WEEK 6

Monday

BREAKFAST

LUNCH

DINNER

SNACKS

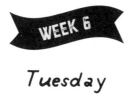

WEEK 6

Tuesday

BREAKFAST

LUNCH

DINNER

SNACKS

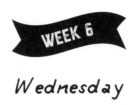

WEEK 6

Wednesday

BREAKFAST

LUNCH

DINNER

SNACKS

WEEK 6

Thursday

BREAKFAST

LUNCH

DINNER

SNACKS

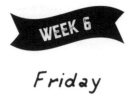

WEEK 6

Friday

BREAKFAST

LUNCH

DINNER

SNACKS

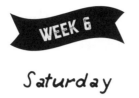

Saturday

BREAKFAST

LUNCH

DINNER

SNACKS

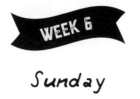

WEEK 6

Sunday

BREAKFAST

LUNCH

DINNER

SNACKS

Microwave
CRISPS

Ohh, man, I love an aul' pack of crisps, crips, chips – whatever you like to call them, they are my downfall! You can't beat a crisp sambo with a pack of cheese and onion, and even a sambo just isn't the same without a few thrown on the side of the plate. They are handy, convenient and leppin' with flavour. These (while they aren't, and will never be, the same as your fave bag of crispy goodness) are a great alternative for a lunchtime snack or a little munch in the evening, and they contain no oils or fats.

SERVES 1

1 large potato (Maris Piper)
sea salt

METHOD

Slice the potato as fine as you can – the bigger the spud, the bigger the slices, but get them thin AF. I use a mandolin; I find this gives the perfect slice with little effort. Then I give them a quick rinse and pat dry with a tea towel.

Pop a sheet of baking paper on a microwave-safe plate and lay out your spud slices, making sure not to overlap them. Pop them in the microwave at high for 7–8 minutes, turning halfway through. They should go nice and crispy when ready. Remove from microwave, pop into a bowl and season with sea salt.

TIPS

Get creative with your flavours – onion powder mixed with savoury yeast flakes makes a good cheese and onion option. If you find yours are sticking to the baking paper, you can spray a little oil on them. Alternatively, crunch up some baking paper, pop this on the plate and lay your slices on top and around it. This will elevate them and help them cook quicker.

Eat in moderation or alongside a main meal. They are still carbs, at the end of the day, and even if your plan says you can eat all the spuds you like, a bit of cop on is required here! You would be likely to eat more of these than you would spuds with your dinner, so just mind yourself and, like everything, moderation.

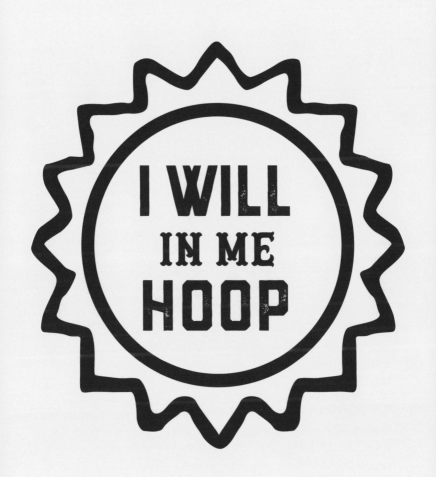

SUMMARY

_____

_____

_____

_____

_____

_____

_____

_____

_____

_____

_____

_____

_____

_____

_____

_____

_____

_____

_____

_____

_____

_____

_____

_____

SUMMARY

WHEN IN DOUBT, LASH IN

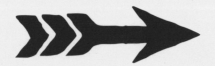

A LITTLE EXTRA
EXTRA
FOR THE
CRAIC

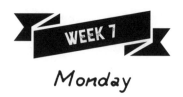

Monday

BREAKFAST

LUNCH

DINNER

SNACKS

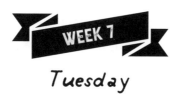

Tuesday

BREAKFAST

LUNCH

DINNER

SNACKS

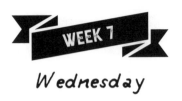

WEEK 7

Wednesday

BREAKFAST

LUNCH

DINNER

SNACKS

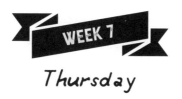

WEEK 7

Thursday

BREAKFAST

LUNCH

DINNER

SNACKS

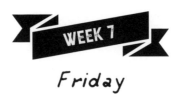

WEEK 7

Friday

BREAKFAST

LUNCH

DINNER

SNACKS

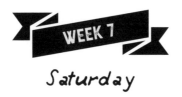

WEEK 7

Saturday

BREAKFAST

LUNCH

DINNER

SNACKS

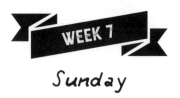

Sunday

BREAKFAST

LUNCH

DINNER

SNACKS

Breakfast
BURRITO

Burritos aren't just for dinner, nope! They are for breakfast, lunch and dinner around here! Put your own spin on it and make these little beauts for a warm hug of a breakfast. If you don't want to add sauce, lash in a few beans to make it a saucy beast.

SERVES 2

4 bacon medallions

2-3 cherry tomatoes

3-4 mushrooms

2 eggs

2 wholemeal wraps

20g grated Cheddar cheese

squizz of BBQ sauce or some beans

METHOD

First, throw your bacon, cherry tomatoes and mushrooms under the grill or pop in the airfryer at 190°C until cooked to your liking. Then scramble your eggs.

Lay out your wrap and add a sprinkle of Cheddar down the middle. Add in your scrambled egg, cooked bacon, tomatoes and mushrooms, and a drizzle of BBQ (or your fave sauce) or add some beans.

To wrap, tuck in the ends and wrap it up so nothing falls out. Pop it on a warm pan, folded side down, as this will seal it when you flip it over. Leave it for 1–2 minutes on both sides – we just want to lightly toast the wrap and make sure the cheese is nice and melty. Cut in half and enjoy every bite.

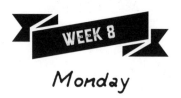

Monday

BREAKFAST

LUNCH

DINNER

SNACKS

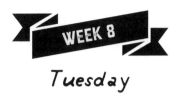

Tuesday

BREAKFAST

LUNCH

DINNER

SNACKS

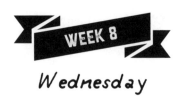

Wednesday

BREAKFAST

LUNCH

DINNER

SNACKS

Thursday

BREAKFAST

LUNCH

DINNER

SNACKS

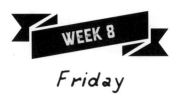

Friday

BREAKFAST

LUNCH

DINNER

SNACKS

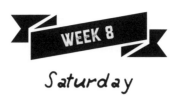

Saturday

BREAKFAST

LUNCH

DINNER

SNACKS

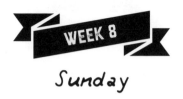

WEEK 8

Sunday

BREAKFAST

LUNCH

DINNER

SNACKS

Cauli Buffalo
WINGS

These masso vegan-friendly (minus the cheese) wings are guaranteed to get those taste buds hopping. So quick and simple to make and absolutely bursting with flavour.

SERVES 2

1 head of cauliflower

25g flour

1 tsp smoked paprika

½ tsp garlic salt

½ tsp garlic granules

50g Panko breadcrumbs

2 to 3 tbsp buffalo hot sauce

METHOD

Preheat your oven or airfryer to 180°C.

Give your cauliflower head a good wash and break into florets.

Put your flour, paprika, garlic salt and garlic granules in a mixing bowl and stir in a little water. Put your breadcrumbs in a separate bowl.

Dip and coat the cauliflower florets in the spice mixture, then dip and coat them in the breadcrumbs.

Pop the florets into the airfryer or preheated oven for 15–20 minutes. Check halfway and turn over.

When cooked, bung them into a mixing bowl, add in the buffalo sauce and give a good mix together to coat them all.

If you fancy a masso blue cheese dipping sauce, see page 247.

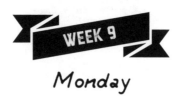

Monday

BREAKFAST

LUNCH

DINNER

SNACKS

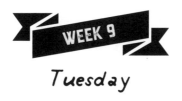

Tuesday

BREAKFAST

LUNCH

DINNER

SNACKS

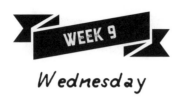

Wednesday

BREAKFAST

LUNCH

DINNER

SNACKS

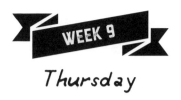

Thursday

BREAKFAST

LUNCH

DINNER

SNACKS

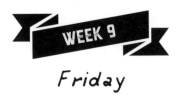

WEEK 9

Friday

BREAKFAST

LUNCH

DINNER

SNACKS

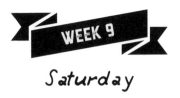

WEEK 9

Saturday

BREAKFAST

LUNCH

DINNER

SNACKS

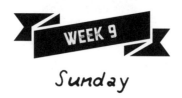

WEEK 9

Sunday

BREAKFAST

LUNCH

DINNER

SNACKS

Chicken Caesar
YUK SUNG

This might sound very fancy, but it's basically chicken Caesar in lettuce cups. It's one dish I always loved when eating out, so I put my own little spin on it. You can create so many different options with these and it's great when you want to cut down on the carbs as lettuce is a nice alternative to a wrap or pitta.

SERVES 2

2 chicken breasts, diced
½ tsp garlic powder
½ tsp smoked paprika
1 head of little gem lettuce
2-3 tbsp light Caesar dressing
Parmesan shavings

GARLIC CROUTONS

½ wholemeal burger bun (for thicker croutons)
½ tsp garlic powder
½ tsp mixed herbs
Salt, to taste

METHOD

In a hot pan, brown off the chicken and add the garlic powder and smoked paprika. Remove from pan and keep to one side.

Chop the burger bun up into bite-sized squares, pop them into the hot pan and coat with the garlic powder and mixed herbs until golden and crisp. Keep the heat low so as not to burn them.

Break off the lettuce leaves and wash them. Fill the leaves with the chicken, croutons, a drizzle of Caesar sauce and a sprinkle of Parmesan. Wrap them up and eat straight away.

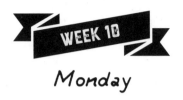

Monday

BREAKFAST

LUNCH

DINNER

SNACKS

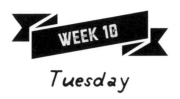

Tuesday

BREAKFAST

LUNCH

DINNER

SNACKS

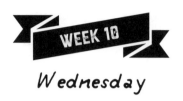

WEEK 10

Wednesday

BREAKFAST

LUNCH

DINNER

SNACKS

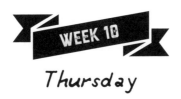

Thursday

BREAKFAST

LUNCH

DINNER

SNACKS

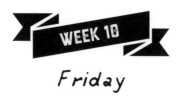

Friday

BREAKFAST

LUNCH

DINNER

SNACKS

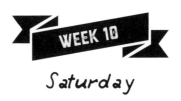

WEEK 10

Saturday

BREAKFAST

LUNCH

DINNER

SNACKS

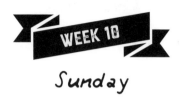

Sunday

BREAKFAST

LUNCH

DINNER

SNACKS

Wild Mushroom
PASTA

Here's a fancy one for you to whip up and impress your significant other, friends or family. Super easy and full of flavour. The main reason here for the wild mixed mushrooms is to give the dish that awesome blend of all the different flavours. The best thing about this is that you can have it done and ready within 15 mins.

SERVES 4

2 tsp olive oil

3 cloves of garlic, finely sliced

1 pack of wild / mixed mushrooms

1 fresh chilli (red or green), finely sliced

1 onion, finely sliced

300g dried pappardelle (or your pasta of choice)

300ml chicken stock

125ml of light cream

60-100g Parmesan cheese

salt & pepper, to taste

METHOD

Get your pan on a medium heat and pop your olive oil in. As the pan heats, throw in your garlic and give it a minute to infuse with the oil and then add the mushrooms as they are (no need to chop).

While this is going on, don't forget to lash on your pasta as per the packet's instructions.

So, back to the pan. Give the mushrooms and garlic a good stir and cook for a couple of minutes before adding the chilli and onion and cook for a couple more minutes, stirring as you go. Your onions will start to go translucent and there will be masso smells going on in the kitchen.

At this point, get your stock, cream and Parmesan and add them all in, keeping the pan on a medium heat for a further 5 to 6 mins.

If you find after this that your sauce doesn't seem thick enough, don't panic – you can add a ½ teaspoon of cornflour with a drop of water to thicken it up.

When the pasta is cooked, drain it off and add directly to the pan, mixing it all together. Serve up and enjoy.

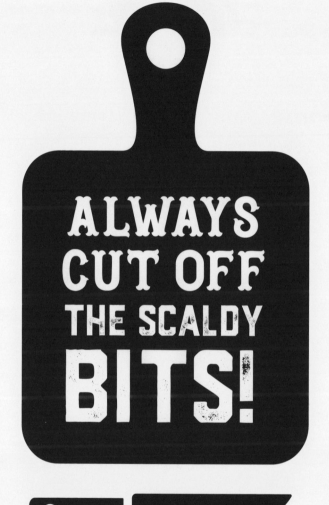

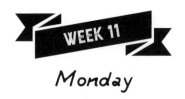

Monday

BREAKFAST

LUNCH

DINNER

SNACKS

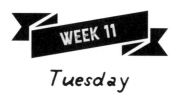

WEEK 11

Tuesday

BREAKFAST

LUNCH

DINNER

SNACKS

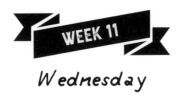

Wednesday

BREAKFAST

LUNCH

DINNER

SNACKS

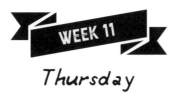

Thursday

BREAKFAST

LUNCH

DINNER

SNACKS

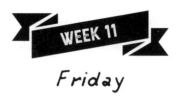

WEEK 11

Friday

BREAKFAST

LUNCH

DINNER

SNACKS

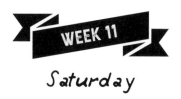

Saturday

BREAKFAST

LUNCH

DINNER

SNACKS

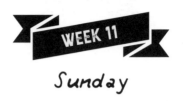

WEEK 11

Sunday

BREAKFAST

LUNCH

DINNER

SNACKS

Easy

SATAY SAUCE

One of our absolute favourite sauces is satay. I'm not gonna lie, this is a little bit epic, lads. You can use this sauce with a dish or pour it over some homemade chips and enjoy.

SERVES 4

2 tbsp dark soy sauce

1 can of Coke Zero

1-2 tbsp of peanut butter

1-2 tbsp of curry powder (sauce mix, not spice)

1 tsp garlic granules

chilli flakes (as much or little as you like)

½ tsp ground ginger

3-4 drops of Worcestershire sauce

salt, to taste

METHOD

Get the heat on under that wok and then add the soy sauce, keeping it on a medium heat. Bung everything else into the wok and bring to the boil until it thickens, stirring as you go.

That's it – you've got an epic satay sauce to enjoy.

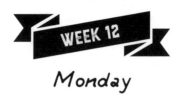

Monday

BREAKFAST

LUNCH

DINNER

SNACKS

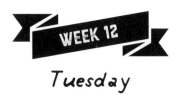

Tuesday

BREAKFAST

LUNCH

DINNER

SNACKS

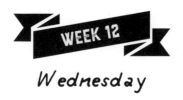

WEEK 12

Wednesday

BREAKFAST

LUNCH

DINNER

SNACKS

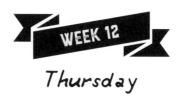

Thursday

BREAKFAST

LUNCH

DINNER

SNACKS

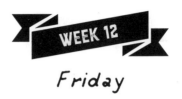

WEEK 12

Friday

BREAKFAST

LUNCH

DINNER

SNACKS

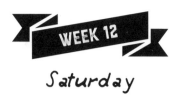

WEEK 12

Saturday

BREAKFAST

LUNCH

DINNER

SNACKS

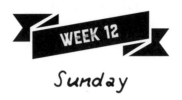

Sunday

BREAKFAST

LUNCH

DINNER

SNACKS

Crunchy
CORN SNACKS

We all know that feeling – you just want a nibble, just a little taste of sweetness, y'know. That little something that will curb the craving or even a handy snack to graze on when watching a movie. These little nibbles will hit the spot and only take you 10 minutes to make.

SERVES 2

large tin of sweetcorn, drained
low-calorie spray oil
twist of salt to taste

METHOD

If using the oven, preheat to 200°C and lay out the corn on a baking sheet. Bake until golden, turning halfway through.

If using an airfryer, spray the corn with a little oil and cook for 10 minutes at 190°C. Keep an eye on them as some airfryers cook quicker than others. Shake halfway through.

Once cooked, serve with a little twist of salt and enjoy this super handy sweet and salty snack.

SUMMARY

SUMMARY

A
SHIT DAY
DOESN'T
HAVE TO BE A
SHITTY
WEEK.

IF YOU
ENJOYED IT,
IT WASN'T
THAT
SHIT
AFTER ALL.

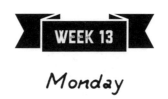

WEEK 13

Monday

BREAKFAST

LUNCH

DINNER

SNACKS

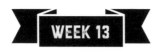

WEEK 13

Tuesday

BREAKFAST

LUNCH

DINNER

SNACKS

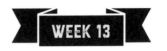

WEEK 13

Wednesday

BREAKFAST

LUNCH

DINNER

SNACKS

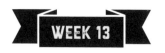

WEEK 13

Thursday

BREAKFAST

LUNCH

DINNER

SNACKS

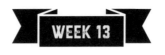

WEEK 13

Friday

BREAKFAST

LUNCH

DINNER

SNACKS

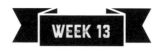

Saturday

BREAKFAST

LUNCH

DINNER

SNACKS

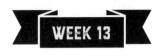

Sunday

BREAKFAST

LUNCH

DINNER

SNACKS

French Toast with Caramelised Air fried
BANANAS

Eggy bread or French toast or whatever you like to call it – either way, it's bleedin' masso and a staple in our gaff and one the kids love to get involved in. Traditionally, French toast is served with powdered sugar, but we like ours with a twist of salt, a drizzle of maple syrup and some fruit on the side.

SERVES 1

1 ripe banana
2 eggs
salt and pepper, to taste
2 slices wholemeal bread
low-calorie spray oil

TO SERVE

maple syrup
fresh raspberries

METHOD

Slice the banana into 1 cm slices. Pop in the airfryer with a light spray of oil at 190°C for 5–6 minutes or until golden. Turn and repeat on the other side. Once cooked, leave in the airfryer to keep warm.

Crack the eggs into a wide-bottomed bowl, add a pinch of salt and pepper and whisk. Dip your bread into the egg, turning to cover both sides.

Pop your eggy bread onto a hot non-stick pan. Turn down to a medium heat and allow to sizzle until golden. Flip over and repeat on the other side.

When ready, pop onto a plate with your caramelised bananas. Serve with a twist of salt, a little drizzle of maple syrup and fresh raspberries.

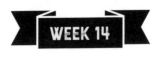

Monday

BREAKFAST

LUNCH

DINNER

SNACKS

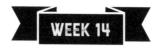

Tuesday

BREAKFAST

LUNCH

DINNER

SNACKS

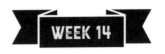

WEEK 14

Wednesday

BREAKFAST

LUNCH

DINNER

SNACKS

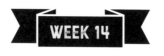

Thursday

BREAKFAST

LUNCH

DINNER

SNACKS

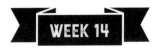

WEEK 14

Friday

BREAKFAST

LUNCH

DINNER

SNACKS

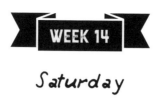

WEEK 14

Saturday

BREAKFAST

LUNCH

DINNER

SNACKS

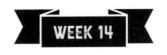

WEEK 14

Sunday

BREAKFAST

LUNCH

DINNER

SNACKS

Faux Pulled Pork
TOASTIE

Pulled pork is fab, but when you want a quick sambo and haven't got the time, this will be sure to get the taste buds leppin'! It's also fab loaded on a pizza wrap or lashed on a fresh batch of homemade chips with some cheesy goodness cheese sauce (see page 73).

SERVES 1

2–3 slices of deli ham

1 tbsp BBQ sauce

low-calorie spray oil

2 slices wholemeal bread

30g Cheddar cheese, grated

tomato, sliced

spring onion, sliced

METHOD

Finely slice or shred the slices of ham and pop on a warm, wide pan. Add the BBQ sauce and coat fully. Remove from the pan and put to one side.

Clean the pan and spray with a little oil. Place your first slice of bread down, add the cheese, the faux pulled pork, tomatoes and spring onion, then pop the second slice of bread on top.

Heat on a medium heat for 3–4 minutes until the bread is toasted. Spray the top slice with a little oil and flip over and repeat so the cheese melts really nicely.

Remove from pan, cut in half and enjoy.

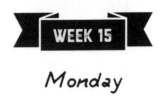

Monday

BREAKFAST

LUNCH

DINNER

SNACKS

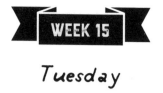

WEEK 15

Tuesday

BREAKFAST

LUNCH

DINNER

SNACKS

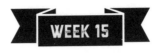

Wednesday

BREAKFAST

LUNCH

DINNER

SNACKS

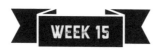

Thursday

BREAKFAST

LUNCH

DINNER

SNACKS

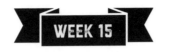

Friday

BREAKFAST

LUNCH

DINNER

SNACKS

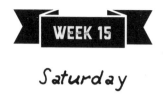

WEEK 15

Saturday

BREAKFAST

LUNCH

DINNER

SNACKS

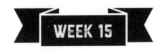

Sunday

BREAKFAST

LUNCH

DINNER

SNACKS

Satay

NOODLE SALAD

When a bowl of lettuce just won't cut it, this noodle salad will get you through to dinnertime, and it will be something you will make over and over again. You can use leftover chicken or make it a little bit more masso and make your own crispy chicken (see page 48, *The Daly Dish*), or you can even use a pack of sliced pre-cooked chicken breasts. Top tip: make a big batch of satay sauce and keep in an airtight jar in the fridge for up to five days – a super timesaver for dinner or these deadly salads.

SERVES 2

fine egg noodles (2 slabs)
2 tbsp soy sauce
sesame seeds, to taste
2 breasts chicken
iceberg lettuce, finely sliced
½ carrot, grated or finely sliced
2 spring onions, sliced
satay sauce (see page 129)

METHOD

Pop your noodles in boiling water and cook as per the packet's instructions.

When ready, throw them in a warm pan with the soy sauce and coat, then sprinkle with a pinch of sesame seeds.

Add in the chicken, lettuce, carrot and spring onion and pour on some satay sauce (as much as you like) and toss it all up.

Serve in a bowl with an extra garnish of sesame seeds.

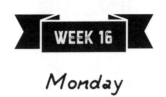

WEEK 16

Monday

BREAKFAST

LUNCH

DINNER

SNACKS

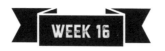

WEEK 16

Tuesday

BREAKFAST

LUNCH

DINNER

SNACKS

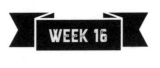

WEEK 16

Wednesday

BREAKFAST

LUNCH

DINNER

SNACKS

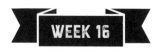

WEEK 16

Thursday

BREAKFAST

LUNCH

DINNER

SNACKS

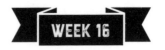

WEEK 16

Friday

BREAKFAST

LUNCH

DINNER

SNACKS

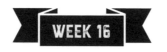

WEEK 16

Saturday

BREAKFAST

LUNCH

DINNER

SNACKS

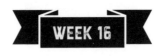

WEEK 16

Sunday

BREAKFAST

LUNCH

DINNER

SNACKS

Loaded Sweet
POTATO FRIES

I love the term loaded fries. I mean, there's nothing better than homemade fries loaded up with some awesome toppings. It makes a great meal in itself or is also perfect as a side dish. It feels really indulgent, but you can make it a lot healthier than you would get from a takeout.

SERVES 2

4 decent-sized sweet potatoes

low-calorie spray oil

½ tsp of cayenne pepper*

½ tsp of garlic powder

½ tsp of onion salt

salt and pepper, to taste

6 slices of Parma ham

50g Cheddar cheese, grated

*cayenne pepper can give you a good kick up the arse, so if you're less adventurous you can use less.

METHOD

Get those spuds and give them a good wash and scrub, getting them nice and clean. We're gonna leave the skin on for this recipe. Get a good strong knife and chop them into chips or wedges.

Once they're all chopped up, pop them into a microwave-safe bowl and whack on high for around 5 minutes. Take them out and give them a good shake about halfway through. The reason we're microwaving them first is to soften them up before we cook them.

Next up, give the fries a couple of sprays of oil, lightly coating them. Then add your cayenne pepper, garlic powder and onion salt (you can also add a little salt and pepper here too if you want). Get your hands in there and gently rub them all together to coat evenly.

Pop them into the airfryer at 180°C for around 14 minutes. Give them a shake halfway through and keep an eye on them so they don't burn – you can lower the temp towards the end if needs be. For oven cooking, pop them on a baking tray and into a preheated oven at 180°C for the same time, checking halfway and giving a shake to turn them over.

While the fries are cooking, get your Parma ham and tear it into strips. Once the fries are ready, put them into two serving bowls, put the ham on top then sprinkle the cheese over. Pop them under the grill for a minute until the cheese starts to melt.

Serve up and enjoy.

WHEN YOU
PASS A MIRROR,
DON'T LOOK AWAY.
LOOK AT YOURSELF AND SAY,

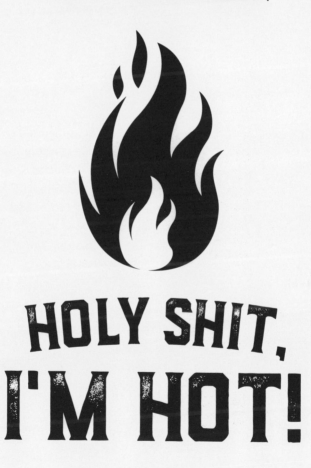

HOLY SHIT,
I'M HOT!

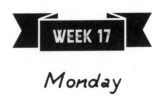

WEEK 17

Monday

BREAKFAST

LUNCH

DINNER

SNACKS

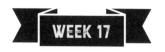

WEEK 17

Tuesday

BREAKFAST

LUNCH

DINNER

SNACKS

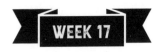

Wednesday

BREAKFAST

LUNCH

DINNER

SNACKS

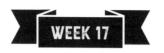

WEEK 17

Thursday

BREAKFAST

LUNCH

DINNER

SNACKS

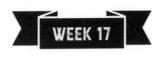

WEEK 17

Friday

BREAKFAST

LUNCH

DINNER

SNACKS

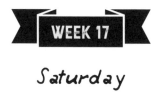

WEEK 17

Saturday

BREAKFAST

LUNCH

DINNER

SNACKS

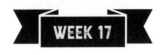

WEEK 17

Sunday

BREAKFAST

LUNCH

DINNER

SNACKS

Easy Sweet and Sour
SAUCE

SERVES 2

3 tbsp ketchup

2 tbsp light soy sauce

5 tbsp vinegar

2½ tbsp granulated sweetener

5–6 drops Worcestershire sauce

5 tbsp of water

METHOD:

Add all the ingredients to a hot wok. Mix well and bring it to a boil, then reduce the heat for 1–2 mins. If it needs to be thickened, mix ½ tsp cornflour with a drop of water, add to the sauce and mix well.

SERVING SUGGESTIONS

Serve with crispy chicken (page 48, *The Daly Dish*), fried onions and boiled rice for a deadly any-night fakemake.

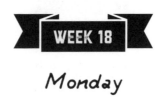

Monday

BREAKFAST

LUNCH

DINNER

SNACKS

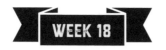

WEEK 18

Tuesday

BREAKFAST

LUNCH

DINNER

SNACKS

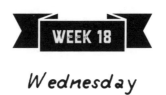

Wednesday

BREAKFAST

LUNCH

DINNER

SNACKS

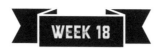

WEEK 18

Thursday

BREAKFAST

LUNCH

DINNER

SNACKS

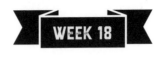

WEEK 18

Friday

BREAKFAST

LUNCH

DINNER

SNACKS

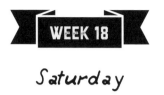

WEEK 18

Saturday

BREAKFAST

LUNCH

DINNER

SNACKS

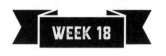

Sunday

BREAKFAST

LUNCH

DINNER

SNACKS

Punchy
PESTO

Who doesn't like a bit of pesto – it was always a fave of mine. This recipe is super quick and easy and you'll have a banging pesto sauce within minutes. And it's so versatile, you can bung it in with some pasta for an epic Pesto Pasta (even add a birra chicken). Or use it as a dip – it goes great with some homemade crisps. One of my personal favorites is some nice toasted sourdough bread with pesto on top, some fresh vine tomatoes, a sprinkle of Parmigiano Reggiano and a drizzle of olive oil – scrumptious. Most shops sell squeezy basil, it's dead handy and can be stored in the fridge between uses, and you can use chopped jalapenos from a jar.

SERVES 4

handful of pine nuts
2 cloves garlic
10 slices green jalapenos
40–60g Parmesan cheese
2–3 tbsp squeezy basil
2–3 tbsp olive oil

METHOD

First off, you gotta toast your nuts! That's right, throw those pine nuts onto a dry pan on a medium heat and lightly warm for a minute or so. You just want them to start to brown (not burn).

Then, pop them into your blender along with the other ingredients. I always give my garlic cloves a quick crush with the side of the knife before I pop them in.

Blend until everything has come together and you have a nice consistency. Serve up as you wish and, most of all, enjoy.

SUMMARY

SUMMARY

_____

_____

_____

_____

_____

_____

_____

_____

_____

_____

_____

_____

_____

_____

_____

_____

_____

_____

_____

_____

_____

_____

_____

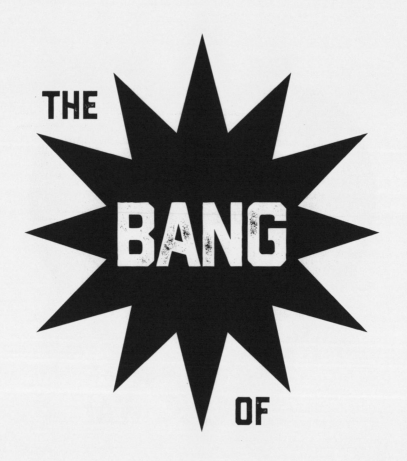

THE

BANG

OF

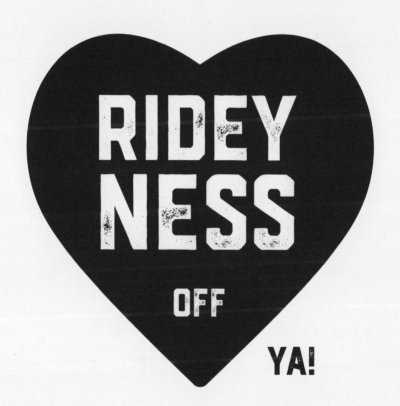

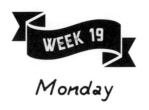

WEEK 19

Monday

BREAKFAST

LUNCH

DINNER

SNACKS

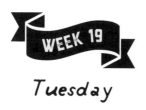

Tuesday

BREAKFAST

LUNCH

DINNER

SNACKS

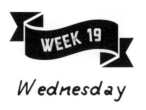

Wednesday

BREAKFAST

LUNCH

DINNER

SNACKS

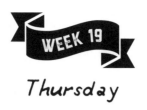

Thursday

BREAKFAST

LUNCH

DINNER

SNACKS

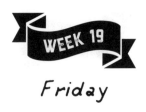

WEEK 19

Friday

BREAKFAST

LUNCH

DINNER

SNACKS

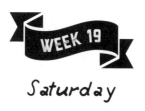

Saturday

BREAKFAST

LUNCH

DINNER

SNACKS

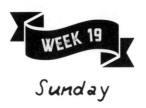

Sunday

BREAKFAST

LUNCH

DINNER

SNACKS

Porridge
BOWLS

I had my first bowl of porridge at the age of 38! Imagine ... It was something that just never appealed to me, and I don't know what I thought it tasted like, but I never even let it pass my lips to give it a try. I eventually bit the bullet as I wanted something filling and quick in the mornings and boom, my love affair with porridge began! It doesn't have to be bland or boring, so here are a few of my favourite combos to jazz it up and it will kick-start your day.

SERVES 1

40g porridge oats
250ml water or low-fat milk

METHOD

Add your oats and water or milk to a small pot on the hob. Keep stirring at a low heat until they start to soften and break down. Bring up the heat a little and if they seem a bit dry, add in a drop of water or milk. You don't want it like cement in the bottom of your pot, so keep adding in liquid until it's nice and creamy. When ready, get creative with the following combos.

TURKISH DELIGHT

rose water (to taste)
1 tsp sweetener
chocolate chips
fresh strawberries

Make up your porridge using the above method and add the rose water and sweetener. Serve in a bowl with sliced-up strawberries lined around the side. Pop in the chocolate chips and let them melt with the heat. Get a big spoon, mix it all up and get it into ya!

MAPLE CRUNCH

1 crushed Biscoff biscuit
5ml maple syrup
frozen raspberries

Make up your porridge using the above method. Serve piping hot in your favourite bowl. Crush up the Biscoff and sprinkle all over the top. Drizzle over the maple syrup then sprinkle the frozen raspberries on top.

PEANUT BUTTER CUP

2 tbsp peanut butter powder
chocolate chips
fresh blueberries

Make up your porridge using the above method. I serve mine hot in a mug. Make up the peanut butter powder with a little water and drizzle in as a layer on top of the porridge. Add in the chocolate chips and the blueberries and you have a delicious, layered mug of love.

IT'S NOT

ROCKET
SCIENCE.

IT'S ABOUT

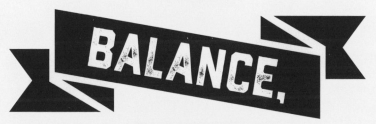

SO DON'T BE

A TICK.

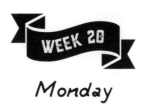

Monday

BREAKFAST

LUNCH

DINNER

SNACKS

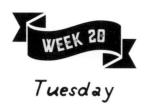

Tuesday

BREAKFAST

LUNCH

DINNER

SNACKS

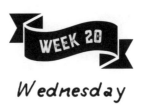

Wednesday

BREAKFAST

LUNCH

DINNER

SNACKS

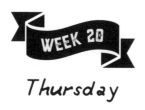

Thursday

BREAKFAST

LUNCH

DINNER

SNACKS

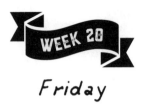

WEEK 20

Friday

BREAKFAST

LUNCH

DINNER

SNACKS

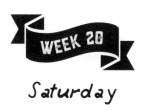

Saturday

BREAKFAST

LUNCH

DINNER

SNACKS

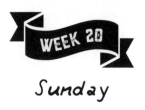

Sunday

BREAKFAST

LUNCH

DINNER

SNACKS

Nacho
SOUP

This is a great way to use up any leftover chicken you have from a Sunday roast or a dinner from the night before, and a deadly way to jazz up that tin of soup that's been sitting in your press. Waste not, want not and all that, and anything for an easy life and a quick lunch.

SERVES 2

leftover chicken
(approx. 200g)

5-6 tbsp buffalo hot sauce

1 tin of no added sugar cream of chicken soup

1 tin of sweetcorn

blue cheese (optional but masso)

2 spring onions, sliced

METHOD

In a hot pan, add your leftover chicken and mix in the hot sauce. Warm through until fully coated.

In a pot, add the tin of soup and warm through. Then add the coated chicken, tin of sweetcorn and a few blobs of blue cheese and finally the spring onions.

Simmer for 5 mins until the soup is piping hot. Serve in a warm bowl.

For an extra crunch, smash a tortilla chip (I like the cheesy nacho ones) and sprinkle on top.

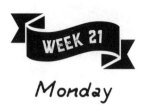

Monday

BREAKFAST

LUNCH

DINNER

SNACKS

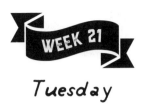

Tuesday

BREAKFAST

LUNCH

DINNER

SNACKS

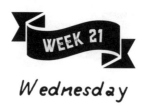

Wednesday

BREAKFAST

LUNCH

DINNER

SNACKS

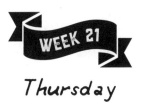

Thursday

BREAKFAST

LUNCH

DINNER

SNACKS

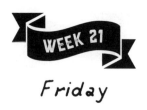

Friday

BREAKFAST

LUNCH

DINNER

SNACKS

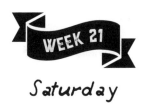

WEEK 21

Saturday

BREAKFAST

LUNCH

DINNER

SNACKS

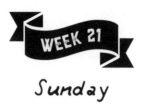

Sunday

BREAKFAST

LUNCH

DINNER

SNACKS

Tuna, Sweetcorn and
PASTA SALAD

Tuna and sweetcorn – always an awesome combo. This is a super quick and easy light lunch idea, ready in minutes and is a handy one to make the night before and bring to work the following day.

SERVES 2

180g dried penne
1 tin of tuna
200g tinned sweetcorn
4 tbsp of light mayonnaise
salt and pepper to taste
Parmesan, to garnish

METHOD

Get your pasta on and cooking as per the packet's instructions.

Drain off the excess water from the tuna and sweetcorn and empty them both into a mixing bowl. Then add the mayo. Mix it all together and add a little salt and pepper to taste.

When your pasta is ready, drain it off and add into the bowl and mix everything together.

Serve up with salt and pepper and a sprinkle of Parmesan to garnish.

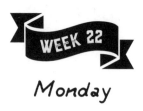

Monday

BREAKFAST

LUNCH

DINNER

SNACKS

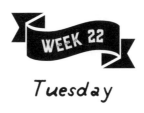

Tuesday

BREAKFAST

LUNCH

DINNER

SNACKS

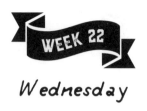

Wednesday

BREAKFAST

LUNCH

DINNER

SNACKS

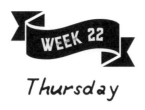

Thursday

BREAKFAST

LUNCH

DINNER

SNACKS

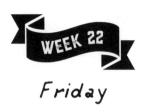

Friday

BREAKFAST

LUNCH

DINNER

SNACKS

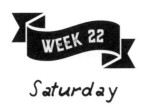

Saturday

BREAKFAST

LUNCH

DINNER

SNACKS

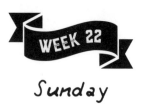

Sunday

BREAKFAST

LUNCH

DINNER

SNACKS

Steak
KEBAB

Ahh, kebabs. We LOVE them and you will love this recipe too. This is a great little hack for making a super tasty homemade kebab without the fuss. You can use all the veg you like and whatever sauce tickles your fancy, but I'm going to show you how we make ours. Now get a tissue ready because you're likely to drool.

SERVES 2

1 tsp chilli flakes
1 tsp cumin
1 tsp smoked paprika
1 tsp dried sage
1 tsp mixed herbs
1 tsp ground ginger
2 lean beef medallions
Use any veg you like, we love:
iceberg lettuce
tomatoes, sliced
onion, sliced
shop-bought BBQ & garlic sauce (I don't mind the few calories)
2 wholemeal pitta breads

METHOD

Start with the seasoning. Mix all your herbs and spices together in a little ramekin or jar. You won't use all of this, so it's handy to store leftovers in an airtight jar for the next time you make these to save you a bit of time!

On a hot pan, add your beef medallions. I cook mine on high for 5 minutes each side as we like ours rare, but cook to your own liking. Remove from the pan and slice finely.

Add a good splash of water to the juices and bits that are stuck to the bottom of the pan. This is going to 'deglaze' the pan and lift off the yummy flavour. Throw your sliced beef back in and coat with all those lovely juices. Then, sprinkle over some of your spice mix and stir again.

In a large bowl, add your cooked and seasoned beef, your chopped veg and a squeeze of the sauces. Toss it all up and get everything coated.

Toast and slice your pitta and fill it up with all that meaty saucy goodness.

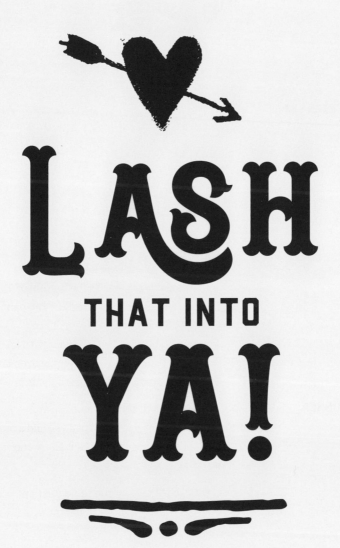

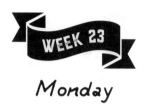

Monday

BREAKFAST

LUNCH

DINNER

SNACKS

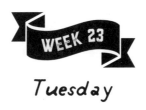

Tuesday

BREAKFAST

LUNCH

DINNER

SNACKS

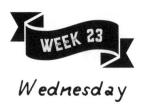

Wednesday

BREAKFAST

LUNCH

DINNER

SNACKS

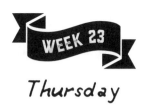

Thursday

BREAKFAST

LUNCH

DINNER

SNACKS

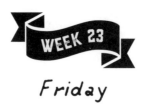

WEEK 23

Friday

BREAKFAST

LUNCH

DINNER

SNACKS

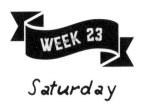

Saturday

BREAKFAST

LUNCH

DINNER

SNACKS

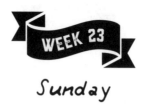

Sunday

BREAKFAST

LUNCH

DINNER

SNACKS

Soy, Garlic, Sesame &
GINGER SAUCE

Let's set the scene! It's Friday night (or any night, let's be honest here – a craving for an aul' takeaway waits for no weekend), and you can't be arsed cooking up a storm. You reach for the phone to ring the takeaway, then you cop on and slap the phone out of your hand because you know that you can make an even nicer version at home in less time than it will take for a delivery to arrive!

SERVES 2

200ml water
½ chicken stock pot
4 tbsp soy sauce
2 tbsp honey
1 tsp garlic powder
chilli flakes, to taste
½ tsp ground ginger
1 tsp sesame seeds

METHOD

In a hot pan, add the water and stock pot and let dissolve. Add in the rest of the ingredients (be careful with the chilli – add a little at first, you don't want to blow the head off yourself). Bring it to a boil and let simmer for 10 mins until it reduces and thickens. If your sauce doesn't thicken, add in a teaspoon of cornflour mixed with a drop of water.

SERVING SUGGESTION

This goes so well with crispy chicken or beef served with boiled rice and lots of seasonal veg.

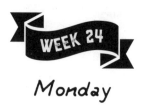

Monday

BREAKFAST

LUNCH

DINNER

SNACKS

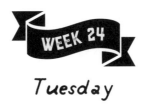

Tuesday

BREAKFAST

LUNCH

DINNER

SNACKS

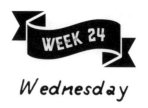

WEEK 24

Wednesday

BREAKFAST

LUNCH

DINNER

SNACKS

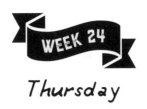

Thursday

BREAKFAST

LUNCH

DINNER

SNACKS

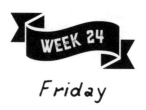

Friday

BREAKFAST

LUNCH

DINNER

SNACKS

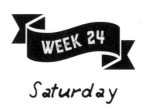

Saturday

BREAKFAST

LUNCH

DINNER

SNACKS

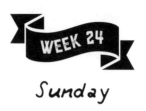

WEEK 24

Sunday

BREAKFAST

LUNCH

DINNER

SNACKS

Blue Cheese Dipping
SAUCE

My love affair with blue cheese sauce began on our travels to the States. I literally ordered it with everything and when we got home it was virtually impossible to find a shopbought version. In steps Gina to make her own!

SERVES 1

blue cheese (as much or little as you like)

2 tbsp light Caesar dressing

METHOD

Put the blue cheese in a little ramekin and pop in the microwave for a few seconds until it melts. Then lash in the Caesar dressing and stir! And it's that simple.

SERVING SUGGESTION

Perfect with homemade southern fried goujons, cauli wings (see page 103), chips, onion rings ... the list is endless.

SUMMARY

SUMMARY

MY MAMA
NEVER TOLD ME

———— ❖ ————

THERE'D BE
DAYS
LIKE THIS,

THE
WAGON!

WHAT I'VE LEARNED

MY PERSONAL TOP TIPS

WHAT WORKED ON GOOD WEEKS

FAVOURITE RECIPES

SHOPPING LIST

NOTES

NOTES

NOTES

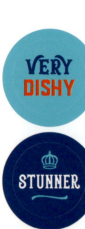
VERY DISHY

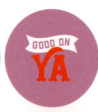
GOOD ON YA

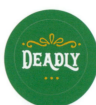
DEADLY

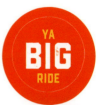
YA BIG RIDE

STUNNER

RIDE

WHOPPER

Deadly DINNER

UNREAL

Little BEAUT

MASSO

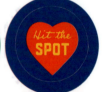
Hit the SPOT

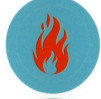

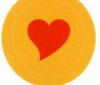

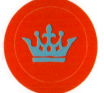

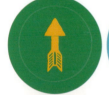

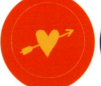

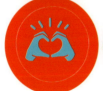

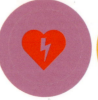

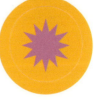

YOU'RE FLYIN'

MASSO MEAL

NAILED IT

A SHIT DAY IS OK

FECKIN' GORGEOUS

GET OUTTA THAT FRIDGE

FAV DISH

BUALADH BOS

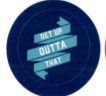

GET UP OUTTA THAT

FAIR Play TO YA

GET YOUR ARSE IN GEAR

STOP THE LIGHTS

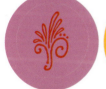

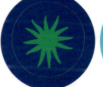

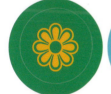

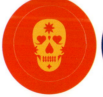

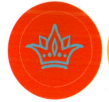

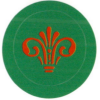